FEEL FABULOUS
EVERY DAY
tips for vibrant good health

Stephanie Tourles

The mission of Storey Publishing is to serve our customers by publishing practical information that encourages personal independence in harmony with the environment.

Edited by Deborah Balmuth and Marie Salter
Cover design by Wendy Palitz
Cover background illustrations by Alexandra Eckhardt
Cover image art © Juliette Borda
Text design and production by Susan Bernier

Printed in the United States by Lake Book
10 9 8 7 6 5 4 3

ISBN 1-58017-889-8

Do you want to increase your odds of living a long, healthy life while staying fit, looking terrific, being socially active, and being mentally and spiritually fulfilled along the way? Of course. Who doesn't? The key to successful longevity, as I call it, is living well every day. It's not just about the length of time you're given on this earth, but the quality of the life you live while you're here.

You must realize and accept that your life as you experience it today is a result of the seeds you've planted in your personal garden. The evidence of these long-life seeds of good physical, emotional, and spiritual health, when sown

in your youth, will be readily apparent as you enter your forties — or even earlier. I have seen the results of many poorly sown seeds firsthand. I know people in their late thirties who partied hearty and neglected their health and appearance; now they are feeling and looking old long before their time. I also know people in their fifties and sixties who have taken good care of themselves, and as a result look and feel many years younger.

Believe me, Mother Nature will have the last laugh if you don't take steps to preserve what you've got. If you're not happy with what you see in the mirror and how you feel, you can, with knowledge and determination, greatly improve these conditions. It's never too late to initiate a change for the better.

Today, there is so much confusing information about how to eat right, lose weight, be more energetic, look younger, de-stress, and be healthier that it can leave your head spinning. I'm here to tell you that it's really not all that

complicated. It's about getting back to basics, back to simplicity, back into your comfort zone, back in tune with what you intuitively know to be right for you. Never forget that you are a unique individual who deserves to look fabulous, live life to the fullest, and feel healthy with every breath you take. You simply can't expect to be physically healthy if you ignore the intellectual, spiritual, social, and emotional sides of your life. Successful longevity demands a life in balance, just as vitality demands a balanced diet. Aging is inevitable, but you can age beautifully, gracefully, joyfully, and more slowly.

Living a long, vital, robust life, and looking great while doing it, is directly related to sound nutrition, proper exercise and skin care, stress management, a sensible wellness program, a feeling of belonging, and spiritual practice. *Feel Fabulous Every Day* is written from the heart, so that all women may feel and look truly fabulous all the days of their lives. In this book I share my secrets — sound bits of advice

that allow me to work a full schedule with energy to spare, stay fit, maintain my youthful appearance, satisfy my soul, and nourish my spirit. I hope they will add years to your life, life to your years, grace to your body, wisdom to your mind, and peace to your spirit.

Blessings to you and yours,

Stephanie Tourles

*"The strongest principle of growth
lies in human choice."*

—George Eliot

Wellness is not something to be obtained from a single trip to the psychiatrist or physician. Being well means being whole, connected — a smooth-running sum of individual parts. A disturbance in one part of your being means that the other components are not working up to par, either. Wellness is the desired end of a multifaceted journey that benefits from myriad ancient, traditional, and modern health-care therapies.

This book focuses on specific ways that you can address present or potential problems that can interfere with wellness and well-being. Try using aromatherapy to relax or energize, learn ways to fight osteoperosis, and master simple techniques for reducing stress. Discover how to boost your immunity, learn to promote good digestion and heart health, find out which preventive health tests you need to take and when, and learn about the benefits of reiki

for body, mind, and soul. Use the information, tips, and techniques given here to improve the quality of your life and make the most of every moment. Go ahead — feel fabulous every day!

Aromatherapy for Body and Mind

True, effective aromatherapy utilizes real, minimally refined pure essential oils that are of pharmaceutical and aromatherapeutic grade. They are often processed from plants that are organically raised or ethically wildcrafted. The practice of aromatherapy has scientific roots. The various chemical components in each particular essential oil have been studied to see how their usage can affect the body

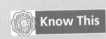

Know This

Vegetable oils, synthetic fragrance oils, and inferior diluted essential oils have an oily texture and leave an oily residue. Pure essential oils are highly volatile, evaporate relatively quickly, and have no oily residue or texture.

on an emotional and physiological level. Many essential oils also contain antiseptic and degreasing qualities, which make them superb household cleansing additives. To guide and educate you in this fascinating mind/body healing modality, I suggest that you purchase an aromatherapy book that outlines the properties and uses of essential oils.

Eleven Basic Essential Oils

The following essential oils have many uses and should be included in the family medicine and cosmetic cabinets. There are dozens more, of course, but these are some of the most popular and the most useful.

• **Clove** *(Syzygium aromaticum)*. A strong antibacterial, analgesic, and antiseptic. It is best known as a cure for toothaches. Place a single drop on the offending tooth and surrounding gum area for fast, temporary relief of pain — then see your dentist. Clove can also be used, like orange and lemon essential oils, in household cleansing formulas.

• **Eucalyptus** (*Eucalyptus globulus*). This deeply penetrating, camphorous oil is a must-have if you're suffering from a head cold or respiratory infection. For relief of stuffiness and congested lungs, boil 4 cups of water, then remove from heat. Add 6 drops essential oil, make a tent over your head and pot with a towel, and inhale the healing vapors for 10 minutes. Be sure to close your eyes and avoid touching the hot pot.

• **Lavender** (*Lavandula angustifolia*). A mild multipurpose oil that smells like an old-fashioned floral perfume. Simply inhaling this oil calms the mind, relaxes the body, and soothes the spirit. This antiseptic healing oil should be kept in every kitchen as a burn remedy. Immediately after receiving a burn, immerse the affected area in cold water or cold aloe vera gel, then apply a thin layer of lavender essential oil. It will assist in rapid skin cell regeneration and help keep scarring to a minimum.

Essential Oil Precautions

Essential oils are highly concentrated natural products that should always be diluted and must be used with caution. To test for potential allergic reactions, try this patch test.

1. In a small bowl, combine 1 or 2 drops of the essential oil in question and 1 teaspoon base oil (vegetable oil or nut oil).
2. Apply a dab of the mixture to the underside of your wrist, the inside of your upper arm, the skin behind your ear, or the back of your knee. Wait 24 hours.
3. If no irritation has developed after 24 hours, the oil in question is generally safe for you to use. If irritation develops, do not use the oil.

• **Lemon** *(Citrus limon)*. Has a familiar clean, fresh, invigorating scent. Use in the same applications as orange essential oil, mentioned below. This oil is also beneficial for oily, acneic skin because of its astringent, antibacterial, and antiseptic properties. Add 10 drops to 1 cup of witch hazel

extract, shake well, and use as a toner to remove excess sebum and residue after cleansing your skin.

- **Moroccan blue chamomile** *(Tanacetum annuum)*. This is a blessing for those suffering from itchy, rashy, dry, or inflamed skin, as well as hives and poison oak or ivy. I like to add 10 drops to a 2-ounce container of skin cream and apply to affected areas as necessary. You may also use this blend as a daily facial moisturizer to keep the skin clear and supple.

- **Orange** *(Citrus sinensis)*. This oil is a great degreaser. You can also add 10 drops of essential oil to 8 ounces of witch hazel for an oily skin toner. Shake well before each use.

- **Peppermint** *(Mentha piperita)*. One of my favorites! Place a drop on your tongue as a breath freshener, or add a drop to a cup of peppermint tea for prompt indigestion relief. For an invigorating, stimulating antidandruff shampoo, add 20 drops to 8 ounces of quality natural shampoo;

Introduction

shake well, then shampoo as usual. It will leave your scalp feeling cool and tingly. To awaken a dull brain in midafternoon, inhale deeply directly from the bottle a few times.

• **Rose geranium** *(Pelargonium graveolens)*. This oil smells like a rose garden. I like to inhale the aroma directly from the bottle when I feel the need for revitalization. The oil has a balancing quality and helps relieve mental stress and fatigue.

• **Rosemary** *(Rosmarinus officinalis)*. The verbenon chemotype is a terrific oil to stimulate your mind as well as your circulation. Add 20 drops to 8 ounces of moisturizing shower/bath gel or body lotion, shake well, and apply as usual. This antiseptic oil acts as a skin-cell regenerative and wound healer and opens sinus passages.

• **Tea tree** *(Melaleuca alternifolia)*. A powerful yet gentle-on-the-skin antiviral, antifungal, and broad-spectrum antibacterial. To prevent or heal infection, apply a drop directly to scrapes, scratches, acne pimples, boils, or insect bites. For toenail fungus, apply a drop to affected toe(s) daily until healed. (Fungus is stubborn and difficult to eradicate. This treatment may take several months to remedy the problem. Consistent application is key.)

• **Thyme** (*Thymus vulgaris*). The linalol chemotype is a powerful — yet gentle to the skin — antiviral, antibiotic, and antiseptic. I recommend keeping the oil around during cold and flu season. Add a few drops to your vaporizer to cleanse and purify the air or purchase a nebulizing diffuser to slowly release the volatile oils into the surrounding atmosphere. Put a few drops onto a damp sponge before wiping down bathroom and kitchen surfaces; it will kill germs.

To help dry and heal pimples, combine 1 drop of thyme essential oil with ¼ teaspoon of aloe vera juice. Then dab on each pimple with a cotton swab.

All-Purpose Citrus Cleanser

Use this general, all-purpose cleanser for greasy hands and dirty bath and shower stalls, ceramic tiles, sinks, or ovens.

- 1 cup soap flakes
- 1 cup borax
- 1 cup baking soda
- 2 teaspoons orange essential oil

1. In a medium-sized bowl, mix the flakes, borax, and baking soda.

2. Slowly add the essential oil, one drop at a time, stirring to incorporate. Store in a tightly sealed container.

3. To use, blend a tablespoon or more of the formula in a small bowl with enough water to form a slushy texture. Use it to wash hands or scrub bathroom or kitchen surfaces. Rinse with water.

Yield: 3 cups

Beneficial Essential Oils

- **Refreshing:** basil, bergamot, cypress, fir, geranium, juniper, lemon, lemongrass, lime, mandarin orange, peppermint, petitgrain, pine, rosemary
- **Respiration:** cedarwood, eucalyptus globulus, peppermint, pine, ravensara
- **Headache and sinus congestion:** basil, eucalyptus globulus, lavender, peppermint
- **Warming:** benzoin, black pepper, cajeput, chamomile, cinnamon, clary sage, clove, coriander, ginger, marjoram, myrrh
- **Stimulating:** basil, black pepper, eucalyptus, lemon, lemongrass, peppermint, pine, sage, rosemary, thyme
- **Relaxing:** benzoin, cedarwood, chamomile, clary sage, frankincense, geranium, jasmine, lavender, neroli, patchouli, rose, ylang ylang
- **Stiffness:** cardamom, eucalyptus citriodora, ginger, helichrysum, lavender, marjoram, rosemary
- **Reproductive balance:** balsam fir, clary sage, geranium, lemon, rose maroc

Aromatherapeutic Massage: Scentual Healing

It's no secret that human touch is powerful. From infants to the elderly and all ages and sizes in between, everyone needs touch in order to thrive. It is reassuring, comforting, energizing, and healing.

For many, the word massage brings to mind pampering, a luxury few can afford on a daily, weekly, or even monthly basis. In this day and age, a bit of daily pampering is just the ticket to unwind from the day's hectic pace. If you have a willing partner, a daily back, shoulder, neck, scalp, or foot massage is guaranteed to put your relationship on a new level and you in a less stressed mood. Self-massage is another option, but I feel that trading massages with a partner is more beneficial. As a treat, try to get a full-body professional massage at least twice a year. Massage gift certificates make a great gift for a dear friend or spouse.

The power of massage is universally recognized, and massage is one of the most widely practiced complementary therapies, with Swedish massage being the most common form. It relaxes muscles (thereby easing aches and pains), stretches ligaments and tendons, and improves circulation (helping to shorten recovery time from muscular strain by flushing the tissues of metabolic wastes). The skin and nervous system also benefit from increased blood flow.

During a massage, the therapist applies pressure to the layers of muscles, generally rubbing in the direction of the heart to promote blood flow. The traditional manipulative techniques can be slow and gentle or firm and vigorous depending on the desired results.

There are many types of massage. Shiatsu, a Japanese acupressure massage, involves work on pressure points. Trigger point massage is a pain-relief technique geared towards particular tender areas where muscles have been damaged or to relieve spasms and cramping. Sports massage is designed to reduce injuries, provide warm-up for athletes before exercise, and help alleviate inflammation.

Custom-Blended Massage Oil

Massage oils can be customized to relax, invigorate, or heal with the addition of pure essential oils. They can be blended to benefit your skin type, as well.

Note: If you are pregnant, avoid basil, bergamot, black pepper, cinnamon, clary sage, clove, coriander, eucalyptus, juniper, lemon, lime, marjoram, myrrh, mandarin orange, peppermint, pine, ravensara, rosemary, sage, and thyme.

¼ cup unscented soybean, almond, apricot, hazelnut, or grapeseed oil for base

Up to 15 drops (if skin is sensitive, limit to 6 to 8 drops) of any of the essential oils listed on page 16, singly or in combination

In a 2-ounce dark glass bottle, combine base oil with essential oil(s). Cap tightly. Shake thoroughly before each use. Use as much or as little as needed to achieve desired "slip" or friction on the skin's surface when performing a massage. May be used daily.

Yield: Approximately 2 ounces

Rolfing involves vigorous deep tissue massage that attempts to align the body segments through connective tissue manipulation, and the Feldenkrais method uses gentle, hands-on manipulation to improve body alignment and breathing; the practitioner also gives instruction on mental imagery and proper movement.

Aromatherapy massage is a combination of touch and smell and provides the ultimate feel-fabulous therapy. The power of smell can dramatically affect the mind and emotions via the olfactory nerves in the brain, which are in direct contact with the limbic system. This integration of aromatherapy and touch is effective for creating a mood or helping to heal a specific condition.

Fighting Osteoporosis

Osteoporosis is a condition of weak, thin, porous bones, and it is not limited to frail little old ladies. Porous bones can be found in just about anyone, from a 16-year-old foot-

Osteoporosis on the Rise

The incidence of osteoporosis is increasing dramatically world-wide, especially in developed countries where protein and dairy consumption is high, rich and processed foods abound, sedentary living is commonplace, high stress is rampant, and environmental chemicals and poisons are encountered every day. Approximately 33 percent of all American women and 20 percent of all American men will suffer serious consequences related to this disease at some time in their lives.

ball player to a 60-year-old man who's been on prednisone to treat asthma complications.

Osteoporosis is often called the "silent disease" because bone fractures and breaks can occur without warning. Often it's the arm, wrist, or hip that breaks. The bones of the spine are also a common area of thinning. Frequently, over several years or even decades, the supportive vertebrae will collapse upon themselves, causing the trademark stooping posture, loss of height, and back and neck pain.

Bone is a dynamic, living tissue. Like your skin, it is in a continual state of flux, always regenerating and degenerating. This constant tearing down and rebuilding of bone helps keep your skeleton strong. Bone health is dependent on more than just calcium intake. Maintaining bone health is not as simple as popping a daily calcium supplement or drinking a cup of milk. Bone health is determined by the interrelationship of circulating levels of minerals, trace minerals, hormones, vitamins, proteins, and other nutrients, as well as regular weight-bearing activities and sunlight.

Build Better Bones

"The causes of calcium loss may include decreased estrogen in women after menopause, decreased testosterone in elderly men, lack of weight-bearing activity, smoking, dietary animal protein, salt, caffeine, and soda pop. In other words, most instances of osteoporosis are due to lifestyle choices," according to Ronald G. Cridland, M.D., certified member of the International Association of Hygienic Physicians (IAHP). Other causes of osteoporosis can include regular use of steroids and aluminum-containing antacids, lack of regular menses, history of anorexia, low bone density, poor dietary habits, hyperthyroidism, and poor health in general.

Osteoporosis does not have to be a fact of life. It can be prevented to a great degree and is often partially reversible with proper diet, exercise, and lifestyle changes. Disease prevention is always the preferred way to go, but it's never too late to take corrective action no matter the status of your present bone health. Here are some tips to help all adults slow and/or prevent bone loss:

• **Strengthen your digestion.** Many Americans suffer from poor digestion. Maximum nutrient absorption is not possible with an impaired digestive system, which tends to get worse as you age. See Digest with Ease (page 46) for a more in-depth discussion of your digestive system and ways to improve its functioning.

• **Moderate your protein intake.** According to John A. McDougall, M.D., "Excess consumption of protein triggers the kidneys to excrete calcium from the body. For people on high-protein diets, these losses are significant. Studies have shown that the quantities of protein commonly consumed by Americans cause calcium to be lost from the body at a rate that is greater than the body's capacity to absorb more calcium. It is estimated that between 1 percent and 4 percent of the adult skeleton is lost each year on the high-animal-protein American diet. This net loss of calcium occurs even when people consume high quantities of calcium."

• **Eat a "strong bone" diet.** Include whole grains, fruits, vegetables, nuts, seeds, canned salmon and sardines and their edible bones, and small amounts of organic chicken, pork, beef, and fish. Eliminate processed foods. A strong, supportive skeleton needs vitamins C, D, and K and calcium, magnesium, manganese, copper, zinc, silicon, boron, phosphorus, and fluoride.

- **Moderate your dairy intake.** Contrary to popular belief, dairy products are not the best foods for building bones. Yes, most dairy products are high in calcium, but they are also high in protein and leave an acidic ash in the body after digestion. This causes calcium to be excreted from the body, not retained. Additionally, after age 4, most people cannot properly digest dairy products because of an absence of necessary enzyme production. Cow's milk is best suited for calves, not humans.

- **Make an impact.** You need at least 30 minutes of daily weight-bearing exercise in order to build and preserve the most bone. Brisk walking, stair climbing, weight lifting, running, dancing, and jumping rope fill the bill. A sedentary lifestyle will rapidly accelerate bone loss.

- **Enjoy a little sun exposure.** I said a little, not a lot! Fifteen minutes a day of unprotected exposure to the sun's rays will aid in the development of vitamin D within the skin, which enhances calcium absorption in the intestines.

• **Don't smoke.** Cigarette smoking can inhibit bone growth, boost calcium excretion, and impair digestion. It also slows the healing of fractured or broken bones.

• **Limit alcohol consumption.** Daily intake beyond a small glass of wine or beer can interfere with calcium absorption.

 Sesame Seeds

The tiny sesame seed delivers a big nutritional boost toward growing healthy bones. This tasty seed is almost 19 percent protein and is richly endowed with B vitamins, calcium, and minerals. Try to find unhulled, whole sesame seeds; these are darker in color and considerably richer in nutrients than their white, hulled cousins.

A good way to add sesame seeds to your diet is to replace peanut butter with organic, crunchy sesame butter. I also like to make sweet sesame snack balls by combining sesame butter with enough whole sesame seeds to form a stiff paste. Add honey to sweeten, then form into small balls, and roll in unsweetened coconut shreds. Refrigerate, then enjoy. Yum!

• **Limit salt and sodas.** Salt and the phosphorus contained in sodas are both calcium-depleting minerals. If your diet is high in junk foods or you eat out several times a week you are probably consuming excessive amounts.

• **Check your medications.** Several medications can increase the likelihood of bone loss. Among these are adrenal corticosteroids (cortisone-like drugs), anticoagulants (blood thinners), aluminum-containing antacids, some chemotherapy medications, antidepressants, certain diuretics, and some antibiotics. Check with your health care provider for possible side effects and how to counter them.

• **Prevent falls.** Practice yoga or t'ai chi to improve balance, coordination, and flexibility.

Stress-Busting Techniques

In these modern, fast-paced times, stress is unavoidable. During times of adversity, your reflexes naturally kick in and the adrenaline starts pumping. Heart rate, blood pressure, respiration, and blood sugar levels increase and muscles tense. The body's fight-or-flight mechanism is in high gear and the alarm is about to go off.

"The highest reward for man's toil is not what he gets for it, but what he becomes because of it."

—John Ruskin

Regain Control — and Your Cool

Before your stress alarm sounds and your world falls to pieces, learn to manage your stress and improve your health by following these tips. Always be proactive in making healthy lifestyle decisions.

• **Be realistic.** You can't be everywhere at the same time, nor can you be all things to all people. Trying to be super-human is a feat best left to Superman. Tackle the most important tasks first and the lesser priorities later. I begin my day by writing down all the tasks needing my attention and check them off one by one as the day goes by. This is very satisfying and gives me a sense of accomplishment.

• **Be aware.** Learn to notice your body's specific stress signals. You can easily tell when your blood pressure is up: your palms are sweaty, chest is tight, neck is tense, stomach is in knots, or heart is pounding. Other signs of stress include difficulty concentrating, general irritability, trembling, feeling "keyed up," sleeping too little or too much, feeling out of control or an urge to run and hide, being easily startled by small sounds, and feeling pressure from within yourself to be constantly productive.

• **Look forward to something.** Plan a mini-vacation, go on a second honeymoon, take a day trip to a historical garden. When stress strikes, recall the event you've planned for the near future and visualize the people you'll encounter and places you'll explore. Just looking forward to something enjoyable can instill a bit of tranquility.

• **Take a deep breath.** When the day isn't going your way, take a breather. Sit down and close your eyes. Press one finger over your right nostril and inhale deeply and slowly through your left. Exhale through your mouth. Now press one finger over your left nostril and repeat the procedure. Alternate this method 5 times on each side. Sure does the trick for me!

"There is nothing either good or bad,
but thinking makes it so."

—William Shakespeare, *Hamlet*

• **Clear up the clutter.** A messy, unorganized home or office instantly stresses you upon entering. I know I'm not as productive when the trash can is overflowing, papers are in piles nearly falling from my desk, and the floor is littered with more piles.

• **Learn to say no.** Eliminate activities that are not absolutely necessary in your life right now, learn to compromise, and by all means be flexible.

• **Get up, go outside, and blow off steam.** Take a brisk walk, ride your bicycle, or play a game of volleyball. The combination of exercise and fresh air will reduce tension, unclutter your mind, ease your frustration, improve your sleep, self-esteem, and well-being, and energize your mind and body. Not feeling energetic? Try a meditative yoga class instead.

• **Relax with herbal tea.** Drink a cup or two daily of chamomile, catnip, passionflower, skullcap, hops, or valerian tea. To brew, pour a cup of boiling water over 1 or 2 teaspoons of dried herb, cover, and steep for approximately 10 minutes. These mild-tasting herbs contain tranquilizing compounds traditionally known to ease stress without becoming addictive or making you feel groggy. They are relaxing and soothing and can help you take the edge off.

• **Good nutrition makes a difference.** Be sure your diet includes the full complex of B vitamins — the antistress vitamins — and plenty of antioxidants. Limit your intake of caffeine and alcohol, which disturb sleep patterns, deplete your sources of vitamins C and B complex, and give you the jitters.

• **Indulge in a stress-reducing massage.** By massaging the area immediately to either side of the spinal column the therapist can stimulate an acid toxin release from the tense muscles, resulting in simultaneous relaxation for the body and psyche. Ask for a massage combined with aromatherapy or an Ayurvedic scalp massage, if available.

• **Laugh!** Laughter is physiologically stress relieving because it can deepen breathing, oxygenate the blood, and ease muscle tension. I love watching a funny movie or listening to a comedian. It's a great way to relieve the tendency to worry and become anxious.

• **"Don't worry, be happy."** Worrying is unproductive and fills your mind with unnecessary, time-consuming thoughts that limit your ability to enjoy living. Instead, focus on a project or hobby that gives you great satisfaction and takes your mind off your problems.

• **Make a change for the better.** Do whatever it takes to erase or minimize the distress in your life. Unhappy at work? Look for a better, more fulfilling job. Fighting with your spouse? Seek counseling. Money too tight? Talk to a financial planner or design a budget. Lonely and depressed? Join a church, go to a gym, or sign up for a new group hobby or activity.

"Every step you take is upon holy ground.
Every moment is imbued with wonder and miracles."

—Susan Smith Jones,
Choose Radiant Health & Happiness

• **Even one negative stress in your life** can cause a serious health risk leading to loss of vitality and longevity. Whether your stress is financial, marital, work-related, lifestyle-related, or familial, talk to someone — don't keep all of your distress and worries to yourself. Explaining your feelings to a psychologist, psychiatrist, or minister may be of considerable assistance in putting your life back into perspective. Don't be ashamed if you feel out of control. Everyone needs a bit of sound, helpful advice now and again.

Develop "Mindfulness"

Mindfulness is the ability to live completely in the present, in the moment, focused on and aware of the here and now. Daily life provides plenty of opportunities to become more aware of both our inner life and our surroundings. "Like it or not, this moment is all we really have to work with," Jon Kabat-Zinn points out in *Wherever You Go, There You Are*. And as Joan Duncan Oliver acknowledges in *Contemplative*

Living, "When we fall into daydreaming and automatic responses, we find ourselves anywhere but here."

Mindfulness is about moment-to-moment awareness instead of scattered awareness. Being mindful helps you group together the distracting bits of information demanding your attention and refocus on the now, the present. By simply allowing your attention to be fully focused on each moment you'll not fret about the future or look back on your life with a sense of regret.

Every day counts. Every hour counts. Every moment counts. Never let the small stuff pass you by. The small stuff makes the big picture brighter, deeper, and bolder! As the old saying goes, little things often mean the most.

Mindfulness-based stress reduction can cultivate relaxation, open the mind to greater insight, improve self-esteem, heal chronic illness, heal anxiety disorders, ease physical symptoms of pain, and enhance health and well-being. This type of stress reduction can include various forms of meditation and the practice of yoga. For information on teachers and classes in your area, contact local yoga studios, colleges, and universities and inquire about mindfulness-based stress reduction workshops.

Need More Sleep?

That's a foolish question — of course you do! Today's adult is tired. It's a plain and simple fact. We're pulled in too many directions, have far too many demands on our lives; something has to go in order just to keep up, and that something is usually our precious sleep. And when we do finally get to bed, many times we find that we're so keyed-up that sleep eludes us. Our minds race, engineering a strategy for coping with the next busy day.

"When sleeping women wake, mountains move."

—Chinese proverb

According to the National Sleep Foundation, though most experts recommend at least 8 hours of sleep per night, adults in the United States get significantly less. On average, working adults sleep only 6 hours and 54 minutes per weeknight, almost an hour less than they're due.

And further, when U.S. adults were asked to rank four strategies for maintaining good health — namely, getting enough sleep, managing stress, good nutrition, and regular exercise — sleep came in a lowly third! Say it isn't so! Receiving adequate sleep should become a priority for us all.

Calling Mr. Sandman

Insomnia is extremely common; up to one-third of the population suffers from it, some chronically. Sleep robbers include anxiety, disease, depression, stress, pain, hormonal changes, poor sleep habits, certain medical conditions (such as sleep apnea and restless leg syndrome), nontraditional working hours, and parenting young children.

As a whole, we are a sleep-deprived society, and it takes its toll on our looks, moods, and health. Sleep is critical to good health and well-being. It rejuvenates the mind, body, and spirit and enables you to function at peak capacity. Here are some tips for blissful sleep that I hope will have you feeling and looking fabulous in 40 winks.

- **Create an optimal sleep environment.** This includes a mattress that offers ideal support and comfort; a dark room (see below); steady, soothing, low sounds like a whirring fan; and a room temperature of 60 to 65 degrees Fahrenheit, which is optimal for sleep.

- **Increase productivity.** Most people shove sleep aside in favor of working more hours with the belief that they're maximizing efficiency, but in fact the opposite is true. You will be more creative, more expressive, and so much more efficient when your brain is alert and oxygenated.

- **Avoid hot, spicy foods at dinner,** as well as caffeine or alcohol.

"Rest, rest, perturbèd spirit."

—William Shakespeare, *Hamlet*

- **Relax before bedtime.** Find yourself too geared up to fall asleep at bedtime? Create a ritual for quality sleep. A cup of hot chamomile, catnip, or valerian (if you can stand the taste) tea works wonders. Hot milk with a dash of nutmeg or a cup of homemade, low-sugar hot cocoa are helpful for many people. You may want to take a soothing bath and soak in aromatherapeutic bubbles scented with lavender, Roman chamomile, or neroli essential oil.

- **Eat several small meals throughout the day** to stabilize your sugar level. If you're hungry and hypoglycemic when it's time for bed, you will have trouble falling and staying asleep.

- **Exercise vigorously in the morning.** By evening you'll be naturally tired. Vigorous exercise right before bedtime can be too stimulating for many people.

- **Wear comfortable clothing** (preferably cotton) to bed, or sleep au naturel.

- **Keep your bedroom as dark as possible** to enhance melatonin production. Melatonin is the hormone produced by the pineal gland that brings on drowsiness and sleep. Even small amounts of light entering your bedroom can interrupt its production, so pull the shades, turn off the television, and put the nightlight in the bathroom. If you must, wear a sleep mask.

- **Go to bed by 10 P.M.** Generally, the more sleep you receive before midnight, the better you'll feel the next morning.

- **Don't work or discuss work in the bedroom.** It's too distracting.

- **Give yourself a nice foot or hand massage** just before you go to sleep. Even better, offer to give your significant other a brief (or not-so-brief!) massage if he or she will return the favor.

• **Once in bed, lie on your back,** close your eyes, place your arms by your sides, and take long, deep, easy breaths through your nose; then slowly exhale through the mouth. Let your mind focus only on your breathing. This exercise almost always lures me into a deep, sound sleep.

Boost Your Immunity

There is much talk today about immune system breakdown and the need to protect the immune system and maintain its strength and functioning. The term immune means to be protected from something harmful or disagreeable. This system is your first and often best line of defense against the onslaught of "foreign" invaders such as harmful bacteria, viruses, parasites, fungi, yeasts, germs, environmental chemicals, insect bites, foreign particles (such as splinters), or even a simple paper cut.

Your immune system works 24 hours a day largely unnoticed — that is, until something invades your body or the system fails. If a mosquito bites you, your skin swells, itches, and reddens. That's your immune system at work attempting to rid your body of the poison. A splinter may cause similar swelling, or even an infection.

"Look to your health; and if you have it . . .
value it next to a good conscience; for health is the
second blessing that we mortals are capable of;
a blessing that money cannot buy."

—Isaac Walton, *The Compleat Angler*

When a harmful bacteria or virus enters your system and your immune system attempts to fight it off, a cold or flu may develop. Most harmful invaders are stopped in their tracks before they have a chance to take hold in your body, but if the immune system is weakened, all manner of problems can develop, such as bronchitis, pneumonia, chronic fatigue syndrome, mononucleosis, cancer, lupus, *Candida albicans* infection, herpes, staphylococcus and streptococcus infections, and arthritis.

With age, unfortunately, comes the increased risk of decreased immunity. Some common problems can include slowed wound healing; autoimmune disorders such as multiple sclerosis, Graves disease, diabetes mellitus, and rheumatoid arthritis; increased infection risk; and cancer.

The key to boosting your immune system is simple. Give it what it needs by feeding it the appropriate fuels: organic, whole foods, immune-boosting herbs, purified water, fresh air, and exercise. Be sure to balance work with rest, maintain a zest for living, control your stress level, engage in a soul-satisfying spiritual practice, and maintain loving relationships.

The Herbal Immune Tincture (see recipe on pages 44–45) can help enhance your immune system when its help is most needed.

Herbal Immune Tincture

This herbal formula is designed to enhance immune system functioning and boost memory and mental awareness, and it is simple to make. All herbs are in dried form.

- 3 tablespoons osha root *(Ligusticum porteri)*
- 2 tablespoons St.-John's-wort *(Hypericum perforatum)*
- 1 tablespoon Siberian ginseng root *(Eleutherococcus senticosus)*
- 3 tablespoons echinacea root *(Echinacea angustifolia)*
- 2 tablespoons astragalus root *(Astragalus membranaceus)*
- 1 teaspoon peppermint leaves *(Mentha piperita)*
- 1 teaspoon gotu kola leaves *(Centella asiatica)*
- 1 teaspoon ginkgo leaves *(Ginkgo biloba)*
- 1 small yellow onion, minced
- 20 garlic cloves, minced
- ⅛ teaspoon cayenne powder or ¼ teaspoon flakes
- 1 sterilized quart canning jar with lid
- 1 large bottle of 80-proof vodka (an inexpensive brand is fine)
- 1 5" x 5" square of plastic film or plastic sandwich baggie

1. On the evening of the full moon, add all herbs and vegetables to a quart jar. Pour vodka to within 1 inch of the top.

2. Place plastic wrap or a plastic baggie over the top of the jar and then screw on the metal lid. (The plastic prevents the metal from rusting.) Shake daily and store in a dark, dry, cool place. Allow formula to synergize for at least 8 weeks, and up to 6 months for maximum potency.

3. On the evening prior to the full moon, strain mixture through a strainer lined with clean pantyhose (so that all fine particulate matter is caught). Press herbs with the back of a large spoon or with your fingers in order to extract all of the liquid.

4. Divide the liquid into several 2-ounce, dropper-top, dark glass bottles. Store the bottles on a dark, cool, dry shelf until ready to use. Your tincture should last for many years.

5. To use, take 1–2 droppersful daily directly on the tongue or diluted in a cup of water. Can be taken year round, but I generally recommend six days on with the seventh day off. Repeat for one month, then take the next month off. Then begin the cycle again.

Yield: Approximately 2–3 cups

Digest with Ease

The adage "You are what you eat" should actually be "You are what you properly digest, assimilate, and eliminate." No matter how healthy your diet, if you can't properly digest your food, then you can't assimilate the necessary nutrients to keep your body functioning at optimal levels.

Your digestive system consists of a 25- to 35-foot-long, winding, twisting tube that receives food at one end (the mouth) and eliminates the spent product from the other end (the anus).

Indigestion is a major problem incurred by a large percentage of the population, especially the over-40 crowd. The manufacturers of popular antacids are quite aware of this dilemma and are quick to capitalize on America's discomfort. Just turn on the television and their ads instantly appear right after lunch and dinner. They offer quick, though temporary, relief to those who regularly gorge themselves on massive quantities of greasy, spicy, or fiber-

Disorderly Conduct

Digestive disorders left untreated can eventually lead to serious problems, such as cirrhosis of the liver, jaundice, hepatitis, diverticular disease, and cancers of the digestive system. Anyone suffering from a digestive problem can attest to how unbearable the condition makes everyday life.

less foods, or those who lead stress-filled lives, smoke, drink alcohol on a regular basis, and eat on the run. If you continually stuff yourself past the exploding point, eat too fast or under stressful conditions, or make poor food and lifestyle choices, your body is bound to rebel.

Guide to Digestive Bliss

Repeatedly reaching for a commercial antacid is not the answer to digestive problems. The answer lies in simply observing the rules of civilized eating and allowing your body's chemistry to do what it's designed to do, ensuring complete, comfortable digestion.

• **Always sit when eating.** When I'm super busy, I find that I often eat while standing and trying to do other chores. This makes for an unsatisfying meal and frequently ends in severe indigestion. I notice a big difference in the way I feel if I simply take 20 minutes to sit down, relax, and enjoy my meal.

• **Say grace.** Offer a few words of reverence or have a moment of silence to honor the nourishment you are about to consume. This simple act alone causes you to pause before eating, thereby putting your digestive system at ease.

• **Give yourself an enzymatic boost.** I find that when I suffer from an occasional bout of indigestion, a couple of plant-based enzyme capsules taken right after my meal really do the trick. Available in health food stores, they assist the digestive system naturally without disrupting the acid/alkaline balance.

- **Eat raw veggies.** Begin your meals with a raw vegetable salad or glass of freshly made raw vegetable juice, such as a carrot, celery, and apple blend. Chew or sip slowly. Raw foods, which happen to be severely lacking in the American diet today, are chock-full of live enzymes that aid in the digestive process. As a bonus, you'll tend to eat less if you fill up on a large, fiber-rich salad first!

- **Eat in a quiet atmosphere.** Turn off the television, put away the newspaper, and eliminate other distractions.

- **Heed nature's call.** Make time to go to the bathroom. By all means, don't hold it all in — you'll just be miserable. Regularity is one of the keys to a happy, properly functioning digestive system.

- **Chew, chew, chew!** Digestion begins in the mouth. Chew each bite until it is nearly liquefied, then swallow. That way the enzymes present in your saliva have a chance to initiate the digestive process. Thorough chewing also promotes slower food consumption.

"To eat is human; to digest, divine."

—Charles T. Copeland

• **Don't eat when angry,** stressed-out, or physically exhausted. Digestive juices are suppressed during emotionally or physically demanding times. Digestion requires lots of energy. Wait until you are relaxed and calm before you eat.

• **Don't drink lots of fluids during your meal.** Sipping is okay, but a stomach full of liquids slows the digestion of solid foods and dilutes the digestive juices. Also, avoid ice-cold beverages; they interfere with digestion.

• **Try to eat at approximately the same times each day.** Your digestive system likes a regular schedule.

• **Don't gulp your food.** Eating behavior that mimics Rover's can cause you to swallow air, resulting in belching.

- **Leave the table when you think** you could still stomach a little bit more. It takes your brain up to 30 minutes to register that it is full.

Love Your Liver

Your liver, which is located on the right side of your body under your lower ribs, is the most metabolically complex of all the organs in the entire body. Explains Dr. Richard Schulze in the May 2000 issue of his bimonthly newsletter *Get Well!,* the liver "Detoxifies, metabolizes, renders harmless and eliminates harmful toxic poisons, chemicals, and substances from your blood. It produces many different enzymes that actually convert toxic poisons into harmless chemicals and then they are eliminated in the bile that your liver excretes."

Your liver does so much for your body that I'd need an entire book to explain all of its functions, but suffice it to say it is vital that you keep your liver healthy for good digestion. To encourage liver health, eat a nutritious diet consisting of mostly whole, organic, high-fiber foods and plenty of purified water. Avoid junk foods, alcohol, fatty and fried foods, processed and chemical-laden foods, smoking, and drugs. Remember, a sluggish, clogged liver produces a sluggish, unhealthy, lethargic you!

Don Ollsin, herbalist and author of *Herbal Healing Journey,* suggests organic dandelion root tea and diluted lemon water as daily tonics for the liver. The lemon water is important for its natural hydrochloric acid, which the liver converts into some 6 billion different enzymes. Dandelion root and leaves are first-class liver cleansers and tonics. Dandelion provides a rich source of easily-absorbable minerals; clears congestion of the spleen, gallbladder, pancreas, bladder, and kidneys; and is rich in organic sodium. It is of tremendous benefit to the stomach and intestines.

Fighting Heart Disease

According to the American Heart Association, cardiovascular disease is America's number one killer. It claims the lives of 41 percent of the more than 2.3 million Americans who die each year. Almost 60 million Americans have some form of cardiovascular disease, ranging from congenital heart defects to high blood pressure and hardening of the arteries.

Exactly how and why heart disease originates in the body is a difficult, complex, and often confusing question to answer. You can reduce your risk of heart disease by becoming aware of your risk factors — personal lifestyle habits and genetic traits that can make you more or less prone to develop the disease. Risk factors such as age, family history, and sex are beyond your control. The major risk factors over which you can exert considerable power are tobacco smoking, high cholesterol levels, high blood pressure, physical inactivity, and obesity.

Four Steps to a Healthy Heart

Reducing lifestyle-related risks yields a big payoff toward preventing heart disease. To keep your heart as healthy as possible, follow these four basic rules:

1. Don't smoke. Did you know that smoking is the single most preventable cause of death in the United States and that the risk of heart attack in smokers is more than twice that in nonsmokers? Smokers, when they do have a heart attack, are more likely to die and to die suddenly than are nonsmokers. Second-hand smoke in your environment also significantly increases your risk for heart disease. The good news is that when you do quit smoking, regardless of how long you smoked before you stopped, your risk of heart disease makes a rapid and dramatic drop.

2. Exercise. Any type of moderate to vigorous physical exercise, preferably a type you enjoy, should be done at least 30 minutes per day. Yoga, stretching, and weight lifting are terrific as supplemental exercises, but you still need to get your heart pounding for a sustained period of time in order to burn fat and strengthen the heart muscle and surrounding tissues and arteries.

3. Stay slim. Overweight is defined as a body mass index (BMI) of 25.0 to less than 30.0. Being within this range puts you at moderate risk for heart disease. A BMI of 30.0 and higher is classified as obese and puts you at high risk. To calculate your exact BMI, multiply your weight in pounds by 705, divide by your height in inches, and then divide again by your height in inches. Note that some athletes and body builders with dense muscle mass may have a high BMI but very little body fat.

4. Eat a heart-healthy diet. Food should be both nutritious and pleasurable to the taste buds. It is not necessary to eat only lettuce, sprouts, and tofu on a slab of flavorless bran bread in order to keep your heart healthy. Choose foods that delight both your palate and your heart, and you'll feel the benefits every day.

Preventive Health Measures: Screening Tests

Quite often, especially if you're under 50 years of age and feeling robust and healthy, the thought of scheduling a visit to your health practitioner for a routine screening test is dismissed as unnecessary. But routine physicals for healthy people quite often include a screening test or two that can spot potential diseases at an early, yet still curable stage, prior to any noticeable symptoms. Screening tests can also rule out a disease for which you are potentially at risk because of either family medical history or exposure to outside influences.

How often should you have the various health screenings performed? There are general rules to follow, but your health-care practitioner should make individualized recommendations based on your present health, family medical history, and other factors (such as prescription medication intake, involvement with recreational drugs, exposure to workplace chemicals, and smoking habits).

The following is a list of periodic medical tests you should have even when you're in perfect health. These guidelines are based largely on recommendations from the American Cancer Society and U.S. Preventive Services Task Force.

- **Blood pressure:** Every 2 years after age 18 if readings are normal, or as recommended by health practitioner.
- **Bone density scan** (dual energy x-ray absorptiometry, or DEXA): A scan of spinal, hip, and forearm bone density at first sign of menopause or earlier if there is a family history of osteoporosis, history of broken bones, past or present intake of prescription corticosteroids, or history of hyperthyroidism or hyperparathyroidism.
- **Dental checkup:** Annually.
- **Eye exam:** Every 3 to 5 years; more often after age 50.
- **Cholesterol test** (serum lipid profile): Once while in 20s, then at least every 5 years or as recommended.
- **Digital rectal exam:** At age 50 or earlier if at risk.
- **Colonoscopy:** Every 5 to 10 years after age 50.

- **Fecal occult blood test** (FOBT): Every 1 to 2 years after age 50.
- **Flexible sigmoidoscopy:** Every 3 to 5 years after age 50.
- **Mammogram:** Baseline mammogram between ages 35 and 39, then a regular mammogram every 2 years between ages 40 and 49, and then annually from age 50 on.
- **Clinical breast exam:** Every 3 years starting at age 20 and annually after age 40.
- **Breast self-exam:** Monthly.
- **Pap test or smear:** Annually after age 18.
- **Pelvic exam:** Annually after age 18.
- **Skin cancer check:** Preferably by a dermatologist; annually after 50 or earlier if at risk.
- **Skin self-exam:** Monthly.

Reiki: Hands-on Healing

Reiki, pronounced (RAY-kee), is a traditional art of physical, emotional, and spiritual healing that draws its name from the Japanese characters *rei,* meaning spirit or God-consciousness, and *ki,* meaning life-force energy. This form of energetic healing bases its theory on ancient Tibetan healing techniques that were rediscovered in the mid-1800s by Dr. Mikao Usui, a Japanese Buddhist.

Reiki operates on the theory that the universal life energy, which permeates all living things, can be channeled through the body via the natural energy pathways — the chakras, nadis, and meridians — and the aura surrounding the body. This channeling releases any energy blockages, allowing the natural life force to increase or balance. The result is enhanced well-being.

What to Expect

During a typical 60- to 90-minute healing session, the reiki practitioner will have you lie on your back, fully clothed, on a massage-type table. Next she will place her hands, palms down, in different positions over the body and hold each position for 3 to 5 minutes. During this time, you draw in whatever energy you need from the universe. The practitioner is believed to amplify this energy by placing her hands on your body.

Unlike massage, the touch is very gentle with little or no pressure. If you prefer, reiki can be performed without touching. The practitioner simply places her hands a few inches above the areas she would normally touch. During the session some people report feeling heat or tingling sensations, or seeing colors.

Reiki is a very gentle form of healing, yet can have powerful results. It is beneficial for a variety of health problems, from stress reduction to cuts and bruises, from headaches to low self-esteem, from heart disease to cancer. You don't have to be sick to appreciate reiki; it benefits people of all ages and can do no harm to anyone.

What did I receive from my two reiki sessions? I had my first session in 1998 while in the midst of a personal crisis.

During the session, I felt a sense of complete peace. My body felt very heavy, as if in a deep meditative state. Toward the end I began to feel shaky and weepy. In fact, I cried on and off for the next two days. It was an incredible release for me. A few months later I had another session, and I talked the entire time. I felt light and energetic afterward.

Two sessions, same practitioner, same techniques, but totally different outcomes. I received just what I needed each time.

Can Anyone Learn Reiki?

Yes, anyone can learn to give reiki to themselves as well as others. There are three degrees of reiki, each requiring an attunement or ritual in which the reiki master opens you to the reiki energy, so that you can become an energy channel. Upon receiving the third degree of reiki, you become a reiki master. At this point you are able to educate others and do reiki attunements.

To find a practitioner or reiki master in your area, check out the advertising section of your local alternative healing magazine. Health-food store bulletin boards are a good source, as is word of mouth. Many practitioners do not advertise; they feel that someone with a sincere desire to learn or benefit from reiki will find the appropriate master.

Final Thoughts

By incorporating just a few of these tips and techniques into your life, you will begin to move surely toward better health, longer life, and a greater enjoyment of yourself and everything around you. Celebrate each day, and live each moment to the fullest!

There is no wealth but life.

— John Ruskin